The Diet Guru

Having a Hard Time Choosing a Diet Plan?

Jastin Stephenson

CONTENTS

Chapter 1: What is Diet?

Talking to your friends, colleagues, and family members, you must have gathered numerous diet plans to lose weight or change your lifestyle. The abundance of information you have received is overflowing and perplexing. Even the internet gives away a range of options for diet plans you have never heard of. Every new diet plan you come across seems to be superior and one step ahead in comparison to the last one, making it tough to choose one for yourself. Choosing a diet plan can be strenuous, and that makes you wonder if there is a sure-shot way for you to lose weight so you can just get on with it. Unfortunately, the truth is there is no such thing as a diet plan that can suit all.

While consuming high-calorie food items such as burgers, fries, chips, sodas, ice cream, chocolates, and desserts can be pleasurable to the taste buds, the choices you make now will affect your health in the future. A healthy and balanced diet plays a major role in promoting and maintaining good health, preventing chronic diseases, and aiding in speedy recovery from injuries. Therefore, it is essential to understand that a good diet can be extremely beneficial in the long run.

To help you choose a diet plan for yourself, I have compiled a list of plans for you to choose from, and included the required details so you can easily put together an informed decision regarding what's best for you. However, choose a diet plan that is best for you based on your body type and condition that either helps you shed some extra weight or gain weight to look fuller. Either way, the key to a healthy lifestyle lies in following a healthy diet.

The Meaning of Diet

The true meaning of diet is the kind of food and drink that a person habitually eats. However, with changing times, the meaning of the word diet has slightly changed. The word diet is looked at more as a verb instead of a noun. Now when you hear anyone mentioning the word diet, the first thought that comes to your mind is that person is controlling their calorie intake. The word diet now is more about restrictions and eliminating certain foods from your life. Hence, it is safe to say that the word has been occasionally replaced by dieting, which is perceived as an eating plan that includes various healthy foods to lose weight. These healthy foods add an array of colors to your plate, including dark leafy greens, red tomatoes, pink meat, pale-grey oats, yellow bananas, etc. Consuming portions of each of these food groups provides your body with the required vitamins, fiber, and minerals to keep you active and healthy.

Although you know the actual meaning of dieting, most of you will still be in search of a short-term weight loss regimen to yield results. But let me tell you, there's no shortcut to good health. The results of following these short regimens will also be short-lived. There is a high possibility that you will regain the weight you had lost or gain even more weight than before. It is definitely a terrible cycle, and I am sure you would not want to be a part of it. Losing weight just to regain it after a short while is not healthy. Hence, you need to have a clear understanding and extensive knowledge regarding fad diets and healthy diets.

You can spend years chasing fad diet plans you see celebrities following, but I have a piece of advice for you:

do not follow those crazy fad diets! These diets might be tempting with their short-term duration and faster weight loss results, but I can assure you not only are they difficult to follow, they will probably land you back where you started. Some follow a fad diet to reach their desired weight in time for an event—a prom party, a wedding, or a special date. On the other hand, celebrities need these quick diets to reach results in the short-run for a role where they cannot put in constant work to reach their desired weight category. When you read up about numerous celebrities following fad diets, it might be tempting to try it, thinking it might be the magic bullet to change your lives. However, I will always recommend against it. The famous fad diet, 5:2, followed by Beyonce, received fame and popularity. However, it was short-lived.

Even the perennial favorite cabbage soup diet trend died out soon after it started. On the other hand, a healthy diet is a balanced diet containing different kinds of foods in certain quantities to meet the daily requirements for calories, proteins, minerals, vitamins, and alternative nutrients. Following a healthy diet has multiple benefits, from not having strict limitations about food intake to having various options to choose your daily meals. One such healthy diet is the alkaline diet, which encourages people to eat more fruits, vegetables, nuts, seeds, legumes and drink a lot of water. Following an alkaline diet, you can cut down on your intake of sugar, alcohol, junk food, packaged foods, and processed foods. This healthy diet is not about staying realistically thin, but it promotes healthy weight loss and encourages exercise. The main concept of this diet is to have specific foods that make your body more alkaline and consume fewer calories to keep you energetic, healthy, full of life, and most importantly, feel great about yourself. Moreover, an alkaline diet is also known to help avoid problems like arthritis and cancer.

Every diet expert will promote a different method or focus on a different food group to get into shape. Pay attention because every diet plan will not work for your body, boost your mood, and keep you motivated. Instead, the essential tip for an outcome-oriented diet plan is to keep in check your overall dietary pattern. Based on this, your healthy diet's focal point should be to replace processed foods with real foods whenever possible because ingesting foods close to nature can create a huge difference in your diet and the way you look and feel about yourself.

All You Need to Know About Dieting

Have you ever wondered how dieting works to burn that accumulated fat in our bodies? If we make comparisons, it is similar to how it works with your savings. The fats in your body are your savings, and the calories you consume are your monthly income. So, what do you do when you are not making enough money to pay your bills? Dip into your savings, right? Now let's understand how our body functions. Fat is the energy stored in our body to help us move around and maintain physical activity. So when you are on a diet, you are consuming reduced calories than usual, meaning you are at a calorie deficit. Therefore, your body is now convinced to burn that extra energy known as fat to survive, consequently resulting in weight loss.

Before you start your fat loss journey, there is something you need to know to avoid demotivation later. There is a wicked truth about dieting; most diets work, but most of them also fail. You might face a failure when you end up choosing the wrong diet plan and do not follow it exactly as mentioned. It does not matter whether you chose a diet to improve your look or health or both. What matters is, choosing a path that gives you the results you are looking forward to.

To reach your ultimate goal when following a diet, you need to be consistent in your journey. No doubt, there will be days when you would be tempted to try a new restaurant that opened up in your neighborhood, or you want an ice cream bucket to munch on while you watch a movie with your friends on the weekend. This is not all, there will be several instances that will come along your way, but consistency will help you progress. Staying consistent with your diet is your commitment to do the right thing most of the time and to get right back on the horse when you fall. You need to build a plan that should not restrict your food forever; instead, it should assist you in selecting a sustainable, result-oriented diet that you can continue for the long haul.

Since you are aware that the main agenda of dieting is to consume limited calories so your body can break down stored fat to release energy, but consuming fewer calories does not mean you starve yourself or just eat fruits and soda to go by your day. These kinds of diet plans might work in the short run, but sooner or later, they will negatively affect your body. The smart way to consume calories is to keep in check the nutritional value the food provides you, maintaining your health in the long run. Try to incorporate all kinds of food groups in your diet to keep your body healthy, active and to avoid any health concerns in the future.

Normally, we have three meals a day. To control your diet, you can cut it down to six small meals, but make sure that you are not fully satiated after every meal. And the last meal of the day should be eaten two to three hours before your bedtime. You will find people who just skip meals occasionally without any well-thought-out diet plan or exercise routine to lose weight. It might seem like an easy way out to cut down your calorie count, however, this has a downside – you will feel hungrier at odd times, causing you to make poor food choices. Hence, skipping meals just out of your daily routine is not the best kind of diet that I would suggest.

Moreover, to speed up your process of weight loss,

combine exercise with your healthy diet. Trust me, it is an effective way to lose weight than just depending on calorie restrictions or following diet plans. Exercising has multiple benefits that you might not even know about. With exercise, you can prevent or even reverse the effects of certain diseases. It lowers blood pressure and cholesterol, preventing any risk of heart attacks in the future. In addition, it also lowers the risk of developing certain types of cancers such as colon and breast cancer. So, if your preceding generations have had diseases such as diabetes that might be running in your genes, you can exercise to minimize the chances of it affecting you. Besides, exercising every day also contributes to a sense of confidence and well-being, lowering the rate of anxiety and depression.

Committing to exercising every day can be a real challenge. Try to force yourself in squeezing a quick run or gym session whenever you find a spare moment in your busy routine. Combining exercise with your diet increases your metabolism and maintains or increases your lean body mass, which in turn helps to burn increased calories each day. Therefore, ensure to incorporate at least thirty minutes to an hour of exercise into your daily routine for faster weight loss and to keep your body in shape. Once you get used to this routine, you can increase the timing for improved results.

Exercising every day at the same time gives you the best results. It is because your body is scheduled to that physical activity every day. Science[i] suggests working out in the morning on an empty stomach is the best to burn the stored fat. Remember we talked about how exercise burns the stored fat. That is why morning exercise is an ideal time for weight loss. Anthony Hackney, a professor in the department of the University of North Carolina Chapel Hill, says morning exercise is beneficial because the body's hormonal composition in the morning is set to support the goal of weight loss. If we look at it scientifically, in the morning, people naturally have elevated levels of cortisol and growth hormones – both are involved in metabolism – hence your body draws more energy from your fat reserves. Moreover, research[ii] also suggests that morning exercise may reduce your motivation for food, in turn reducing your appetite throughout the day. So, are you ready to set the alarm early in the morning?

Not Every Diet Suits Every Individual

Have you seen twins in your family or friends? Don't they look similar according to their facial features, but if you notice, their choices will differ. If you present them with the same food, they might not react to it the same way because of a difference in personality. The same theory is applicable for diets – the same diet will not suit every individual. Even though our bodies have the same organs, but the way they function can differ, such as the blood work for each individual is different. You must wonder why your friend can munch on snacks, ice-creams, and soda but does not gain weight? However, if you follow the same diet as your friend, you will end up gaining extra weight. It is because the metabolism, a complex process by which your body converts what you eat and drink into energy, differs for every human being. Metabolism varies depending on gender, age, genetics, and the amount of lean muscle and fat tissue available in the body.

A study was also conducted to research if two people can follow the same diet. An Israeli[iii] study suggests that two people can follow the same diet. Still, only one will end up losing weight since each individual will respond to foods mentioned in a particular diet quite differently. In this study, the Israeli researchers recruited 800 adults to collect their baseline data with the help of questionaries, body measurements, blood tests, glucose monitoring, stool assays and requested the recruiters to track their daily food intake via a mobile application. These participants were then counseled to follow the same menu plan for some time. As expected, the subjects responded differently to the same foods. The results of the study also indicated that age and body weight impacted blood sugar levels after meals. In addition to this, when the researchers fed the same meals with similar glycemic index values to a single individual at different times of the day, the response was quite different to each of the meals.

Another study[iv] conducted by the researchers from King's College London and Massachusetts General Hospital explored how participants processed their meals. Their key findings suggested that some participants showed a rapid and prolonged increase in blood sugar and insulin levels in the body with response to certain foods. Finally, the results also proved that people reacted to meals differently depending on the time of the day and when they recently exercised.

Find a Balanced Diet – For Your Body Type

Now that you are aware of how every individual's body type reacts differently let me try to help you find a balanced diet for your body type. It goes without saying, you need to choose a balanced diet to fulfill your daily nutritional needs. Regardless of their body type, every human needs a certain number of calories and nutrients to stay healthy. Opting for a balanced diet instead will provide your body with enough nutrients without exceeding the recommended daily calorie intake. A balanced diet includes proportions of proteins, minerals, vitamins, fibers, antioxidants, and nutraceuticals that have attached positive health advantages. To sum it up, a balanced diet should offer around 60-70 percent of total calories from carbohydrates, also known as carbs, 10-12 percent from proteins, and 20-25 percent of total calories from fat.

Are you struggling to lose weight even after following a balanced diet? This can be because of your body type. Each body type requires a different diet as well as an exercise routine for the best results. Knowing your body type informs you where and when your body stores fat. This surely has a big influence on your weight and health.

Let me take you through the three basic body types: ectomorphs, endomorphs, and mesomorphs. People with ectomorph body type are long and lean, with little body fat and muscle. Such people have a hard time gaining weight because they have a faster metabolism digesting all the calories they consume and converting it into energy. If we look around, models and basketball players best fit in this category. Many people crave such a body figure, but the ones that have this body type usually long for curves and muscles. Generally, people with ectomorph body types follow diets that will help them gain weight instead of losing weight. People falling in this category should eat more complex carbs, such as brown rice and bread, to keep you feel full for longer and push protein in the body to your muscles to help them grow.

The second type, endomorphs, have lots of body fat, muscle, and their tendency to gain weight is faster than the rest. This is because they have a slower metabolism rate, and their bodies store muscle and fat in the lower half of their bodies. People with such a body type need to have a stricter eating plan involving fewer carbs and higher proteins. If you fall in this category, to lose weight, you need to incorporate aerobic exercises and HIIT (high-intensity interval training) into your exercise routine. For endomorphs, sticking to a keto diet, intermediate fasting, and alkaline diets will eventually result in a healthy weight loss.

The third body type, mesomorphs, fall in the middle of both body types. They can be both lean and muscular and not overweight either. The best part is they do not have to worry about what they eat because they can gain and lose weight without much effort. You can call them natural athletes build with well-defined muscles. That being said, if you fall in this category, you do not need to stress or go insane exercising. Add in a mix of both cardio and weight training to maintain your weight or reach that perfect figure you have always envisioned. If you feel you are on the heavier side, you can follow intermediate fasting for a while for exceptional results.

If you are disappointed with the body type category

you fall in, don't be! Your body type is not a life sentence. It can shift based on your lifestyle, activity, and diet modification. The human body is highly adaptable. If you continue to religiously follow the changes made to your physical training and diet, you can strongly influence improving your body composition. Be mindful, dieting is not for a short time; instead, it is a lifestyle that you must follow.

So, make sure to understand what your body prefers and how it reacts to different kinds of foods to make the right choice in choosing the best diet plan for yourself.

Chapter 2: The Keto Diet

If you have been trying to explore different diets to reach your desired goal weight, I am sure you would not have missed out on the newest buzzword in the diet world, Keto. It is one of those trending low carbohydrate diets that initiate rapid weight loss. Moreover, it is also the most googled food-related topic in the world.

The keto diet is the most popular and trending diet, providing your body with high-fat, moderate proteins, and low carbs. With this breakdown of macronutrients, you body draws most calories from fats and protein and the least calories from carbohydrates. With this, you cut down on most of your carbs such as sugar, soda, pastries, and white bread. Every keto diet variation you come across, will limit the carbohydrates consumption to around 20 to 50 grams per day and filling your body with 60 to 80 percent fat sources, such as meat, fish, eggs, nuts, and healthy oils. Other than carbs, it is also crucial to moderate your protein consumption, because if you consume proteins in high amounts they can also be converted into glucose, slightly slowing down your weight loss transition.

How Does Keto Diet Work?

Normally, the body's cells use glucose as their primary form of energy. The carbs you consume are broken down into simple sugars that are later used either by storing glucose as fuel or storing it in the liver and muscles as glycogen. When following the keto diet, your body is low on carbohydrates, and in this situation, your body will adopt an alternative strategy to meet the energy requirements. The body will start to burn the unwanted fat in the body for energy, explicitly relying on fat stores and glucose from triglycerides.

As a byproduct of this process, ketones are produced in the body. These are acids that build up in your blood and leave the body through urine. Ketones indicate that your body is breaking down fat, and you are on your journey towards weight loss and in a metabolic state of ketosis. Ketosis refers to the metabolic state in which the body converts the fat stores into energy, releasing ketones in the process.

Different Types of Ketogenic Diet

The promising keto diet gives many people increased mental and physical energy throughout the day while controlling their calorie intake since fat and protein can be highly satiating. Hence, you can use the ketogenic diet to help lose weight or maintain it.

Following a ketogenic diet and bringing your body into the state of ketosis can be brought about in a few ways. There is no one ketogenic diet, however, there are four different variants of the diet that you can follow depending on your requirements and body type. But if you are new to this, the ideal way would be to follow the standard ketogenic diet (SKD) for two to three weeks and observe your body changes. Once you are "fat-adapted" or your body has adapted to ketosis, you can try different variations to see which works the best for you.

Standard Ketogenic Diet

Strategic ketogenic diet (SKD) is the most basic of them all. It is essentially the genuine keto diet and perfect for beginners. In a SKD, the diet plan includes consuming extremely low carbs, moderate proteins, and high fats. Overall, your diet should contain 75 percent fat, 20 percent protein, and approximately 5 to 10 percent carbohydrates.

Fats bring in the majority of calories in this diet since it is the primary macronutrient that will provide the body with energy. Following the standard ketogenic diet, many people have shown success in losing weight, improved blood glucose control, and improved heart health.

Targeted Ketogenic Diet

The second ketogenic diet is a significant variation to follow if you observe that a SKD diet hinders your performance during workouts. This diet is called the targeted ketogenic diet (TKD), and as the name suggests, in this diet, you consume small carb-containing meals either before or after your workout. The macronutrient ratio is targeted in this ketogenic diet is 65 to 70 percent fat, 20 percent proteins, and 10 to 15 percent carbs. For most people, adding 30-40 grams of carbs each day pre-workout or post-workout should suffice. But ensure that you are also cutting down on the fat intake by just a small amount to compensate for the added carbs.

In layman's terms, the targeted ketogenic diet is nothing more than a regular keto diet, with just the exception of eating carbs around your workout timings. Hence, each day you exercise, you will consume more carbohydrates. But on days you do not exercise, you will follow the SKD diet. This diet is formulated especially for people who exercise regularly at high intensities or for extended periods. On the flip side, if you are sedentary or perform a low-intensity exercise a couple of times a week, all you need is the standard ketogenic diet.

Cyclical Ketogenic Diet

Lastly, there is the cyclical ketogenic diet (CKD), also known as carb backloading. It is a more progressive keto diet variation that incorporates cyclical carbohydrate refeeds. Meaning there will be some days during the week when you will consume more carbohydrates to refeed or replenish the body's depleted glucose reserves. In simpler terms, you will follow the basic/standard ketogenic diet protocol from Monday to Friday, but on the weekends, you will have a higher carb consumption. The macronutrient in a CKD diet is 75 percent fat, 15 to 20 percent protein, 5 to 10 percent carbs on keto days or weekdays, and on the weekends, it will be 25 percent fat, 25 percent protein, and 50 percent carbs.

The cyclical ketogenic diet is popular amongst athletes and people who seek muscle growth and improved exercise performance. CKD diet is favorable for athletes because the diet plan provides higher carb days to replenish the body's glycogen levels lost from muscles during strenuous workouts. Though researchers speculate that the cyclical diet is superior to the standard version, the variation helps boost the body's strength and muscles.

High Protein Ketogenic Diet

This diet plan entails about 120 grams of protein and 130 grams of fat per day. In this variation, carbs are still restricted to less than 10 percent of the daily calories. This diet's macronutrient ratio is 60 to 65 percent fat, 30 percent protein, and around 5 to 10 percent carbs. Many people have found this modified keto diet easier to follow because it includes more proteins and less fat in comparison to the SKD. The caveat with this approach is that your body may not result in ketosis, because like carbs, your body can convert protein into glucose for fuel. But HPKD will result in weight loss.

Benefits of Keto Diet

As mentioned before, a keto diet's primary goal is to get more calories from fats than from carbs. The Keto diet has gained extreme popularity over the decades, but such low-carb diets have also been controversial. Some people avow that following such ketogenic diets raises cholesterol and causes heart diseases due to high-fat content. However, most scientific studies prove that low-carb diets are healthy and beneficial if the amount of fat consumed is moderated and strictly followed as mentioned in the diet plan.

Primarily, a keto diet's health benefit is to promote weight loss over an extended period of time. Restricting carbohydrates to be in a state of ketosis leads to both, reduction in body fat and an increase or retention of muscle mass. Moreover, according to research[v] ketogenic diet is safe for significantly overweight or obese people. An Australian study[vi] revealed that obese people were able to lose 15 kg on average in a year. Comparing the amount of weight loss in a low-fat diet to a low-carb diet shows 3 kg more weight loss.

If you are concerned about promoting weight loss, you will find several studies that prove low carb diets help to lose weight at a fast rate than low-fat diets. Isn't it surprising that low-fat diets actively restrict calories, yet they are not as beneficial as low-carb diets? Well, it is no magic, but there is science behind this; with a low-carb diet, your body gets rid of the excess water from your body, lowering the insulin levels and leading to rapid weight loss.

Along with weight loss, it also aids in boosting your metabolism and reducing the appetite. A scientific study[vii] was conducted to understand if ketogenic diets support a loss in appetite. The results show that when people cut carbs and eat more proteins and fats, they eat fewer calories than before.

Cutting down on carbs leads to a significant

reduction in blood pressure, lowering the risk of many diseases, such as heart disease, stroke, and kidney failure. A Keto diet lowers the risk of heart diseases because of two main reasons; increased HDL production and reduced levels of triglycerides. Sounds complicated? Read below to understand in more detail.

In our body's cholesterol travels through the blood on proteins called lipoproteins. There are two types of lipoproteins carrying cholesterol throughout the body: high-density lipoproteins (HDL) and low-density lipoproteins (LDL). The LDL proteins are known as bad cholesterol, making up most of your body's cholesterol. Following the keto diet, you increase the levels of high-density lipoproteins (HDL), also known as good cholesterol, in the blood. Hence, the higher the HDL level relative to LDL, the lower the risk of heart disease.

Triglycerides are fat molecules that circulate in your blood, and with high levels of these fat molecules, the chances of a strong heart disease increase. The main drivers of elevated triglycerides levels are carb consumption, especially simple sugar fructose. So, when you cut down on carb consumption, your body tends to experience a reduction in triglycerides, consequently lowering the risk of heart disease.

If you are an athlete and exploring the best diet to improve your performance, you should try the keto diet. Even research[viii] suggests that the keto diet highlights potential improvements in athletic performance. It is due to low-carb diets that allow athletes to rely on stored fat energy during exercise rather than refuel with simple carbohydrates (fruits, milk, and milk products) during endurance training and competition while improving recovery times.

The Keto diet is not only favorable in reducing the risk of heart diseases, but it is also known to prevent or treat certain cancers. However, the keto diet is not solely responsible for curing cancer. According to research[ix] you need to use it along with traditional treatments such as chemotherapy, radiation, and surgery if you are suffering from cancer. Following the diet and the treatments is because it will help in causing oxidative stress in cancer cells than normal cells, causing them to die. Furthermore, the ketogenic diet tends to reduce the risk of insulin complications[x], reducing blood sugar levels. In our body, the hormone insulin is responsible for controlling blood sugar levels that may have links to some cancers.

Following a ketogenic diet is found to be supportive for people with diabetes as well. People with type 1 and type-2 diabetes have experienced an impressive reduction in blood sugar levels. In some cases, values have returned to a normal range, resulting in discontinuing or reducing medications.

These are only some of the most common and topmost benefits of the keto diet that I have highlighted. Besides these benefits, the keto diet helps women with PCOS try to reduce weight, for people with Parkinson's disease and Autism disease, and children with epilepsy. Moreover, some say it has also been positive for people with brain injuries or disorders, but no quality human studies have proven this.

Choosing the Best Keto Diet for Your Body Type

There is no denying that the ketogenic diet is the

most popular low-carb diet trend. If you have researched, you would have noticed many celebrities following keto diets. Although celebrities were not the ones to start the keto diet trend, they have certainly added fuel to the fire. The Kardashians, Megan Fox, LeBron James, Venessa Hudgens, Tim Tebow, and many others follow the keto diet. This is why the keto diet has skyrocketed in terms of popularity in recent years. When you see your favorite actor, TV star, or sports star following it, you instantly want to try it out for yourself. However, the keto diet should not be followed just because your favorite celebrity has pursued it. Instead, you should first understand your body type and set a target goal for yourself. Knowing your body type is valuable knowledge that enables you to determine the proper nutrient intake your body requires. To assist you in this regard, I will now build upon the information regarding body types in the previous chapter and which variant of the ketogenic diet is beneficial for your body type.

Ectomorphs work well with a high-carbohydrate diet since they are lean with a faster metabolism than the rest. Therefore, a low-carb keto diet will not apply to ectomorphs who want to gain some weight. Apart from people who love their body type, a cyclical keto diet (CKD) is highly recommended to keep your body type and gain the right amount of nutrients to keep you healthy and strong. This diet's benefit for ectomorphs is that they do not have to follow the diet religiously the whole week and can easily save off days for birthdays, vacations, holidays, and special occasions.

Following a standard ketogenic diet is the best for endomorphs or people with extra body fat and a higher tendency to gain weight. Your meals and snacks will revolve around meats, fatty fish, avocados, butter, and olive oil with this diet. You will have to consume more leafy greens and non-starchy veggies such as broccoli, lettuce, and cauliflower. Following the SKD will help you to shed more pounds and at a faster rate.

If you happen to fall in the category of Mesomorph body type, you have a choice between the targeted keto diet (TKD) and the high-protein keto diet (HPKD).

I would recommend the targeted keto diet if you are an active individual or an athlete who exercises a keto lifestyle but require more carbs to continue exercising.

Following TKD, you can consume 20 to 30 grams of carbohydrates immediately before and after training or a high-intensity workout for enhanced recovery. Mesomorph body types do not store fat because the additional carbs are readily burned off through intense exercises. Therefore, the best option is to include dairy products, fruits, and sports nutrition products in your diet.

With intense training and physical activity, mesomorphs have a high metabolism. Therefore, sticking to a high protein diet is essential to provide your body with enough proteins for tissue and muscle repair and faster workout recovery. You might be wondering this keto plan might not result in the desired amount of ketosis, however, in this diet, protein is used instead of glucose for energy. Thus, this keto diet variation is more favorable for mesomorph body types, resulting in weight loss and muscle repair.

Whether you are an ectomorph, mesomorph, or endomorph, you will indeed find a variation of the keto diet suitable for you. It is important to note that you need to keep track of your food choices and conduct proper research about the keto properties of the food you eat.

What to Eat during Keto Diet

The ketogenic diet has such a high-fat requirement, followers need to consume fat in every meal. For a 2000 calorie diet, your aim should be to consume 165 grams of fat, 40 grams of carbs, and 75 grams of proteins. However, this ratio can vary depending on the type of keto diet you choose for yourself. Following a keto diet can be tricky, therefore you need to understand the food items that you can eat, and the food items you need to avoid.

Let's first discuss the food items that you can consume when following a low-carb keto diet. To reach ketosis, you will have to avoid too many carbs. This means you need to keep the carb intake under 50 grams of net carbs per day, ideally below 20 grams.

Protein is part of the keto diet, so in the meat and poultry category, you can have beef, pork, lamb, wild game, and all kinds of poultry. Even soy products like tofu and tempeh are allowed. Do not be disappointed if you are a fan of sausages and cold cuts because such deli meats can also be a part of your diet routine. However, ensure to choose items with no added sugars, starches, or breading to keep carbs low.

In the seafood category, most fish and shellfish are keto-friendly. Fatty fishes such as salmon, sardine, mackerel, and herring are excellent choices for you. Moreover, mild white fishes, such as cod, halibut, and trout, can also be included in your diet plan.

You can consume eggs in the keto diet as well. Have them boiled, fried in butter, or an omelet for a quick and inexpensive meal. You can enjoy eggs as often as you like since you must avoid carbs but not dietary cholesterol in the keto diet.

Invest in non-starchy veggies during the keto diet since they are low in calories and carbs but high in providing nutrients to the body. Non-starchy vegetables include leafy greens and crunchy salad veggies such as broccoli, cucumber, celery, avocado, spinach, zucchini, and radishes. Therefore, aim for non-starchy vegetables with less than 8 grams of net carbs (total carbs minus fiber) per cup.

Wondering what kind of fruits you can consume, since most of them contain too much sugar? In keto diet you can eat tart fruits, such as berries, lemons, and limes, as long as the serving size is small. The same is true for melons since they have high water content. If you do not want to consume fruits separately, you can always have fresh berries with whipped cream and shaved dark chocolate, the perfect delicious keto dessert. You might have to avoid fruits such as mangoes, bananas, and grapes that give your body an entire day's worth of carbs in one cup serving.

In a keto diet, nuts and seeds are allowed because they are low on carbs. But there are two things you need to consider. First, you cannot have too many nuts, so start with about 25 grams only for a snack. Secondly, it also matters on the kind of nut you choose, so make sure to avoid cashews, pecans, and macadamia nuts because they are much higher in carbs. Instead, you can enjoy pumpkin, sunflower, and other seeds when on a keto diet.

Cheese, butter, and cream are all a part of the keto diet. I would suggest you include Greek yogurt for a high protein breakfast with few carbs. Besides, higher-fat yogurts and cottage cheese help keep you full for longer, and full-fat products are a part of the ketogenic diet. But you might want to steer away from low-fat yogurts since they are full of added sugars.

If you are a caffeine addict, plain coffee and tea are allowed in a keto diet since they contain zero grams of carbs, fat, or protein. If you must have the coffee sweetened, replace the sugar with a non-caloric sweetener. Adding a small amount of milk or cream is also acceptable. There is a unique coffee called bulletproof coffee with an additional fat content from butter or coconut oil for keto followers. You can intake all kinds of tea; black, green, mint, or herbal because all are carb-free. The same advice for tea is to skip the sugar and add a non-caloric sweetener if needed.

Similar to other diets, the keto diet also restricts the intake of sugary foods. Therefore, you should avoid sugary foods such as sodas, sports drinks, cookies, biscuits, cakes, ice creams, and breakfast cereals. Even savory products such as ketchup, pasta sauce, and salad dressings are to be avoided because they often contain sugar. Make sure to read the labels carefully before you pick them up from the grocery store. Moreover, natural sweeteners, such as honey, maple syrup, and agave, are sugars. Hence, you need to avoid them sticking to the diet plan.

Starchy foods and whole-grain foods are also to be avoided when on a keto diet. This includes bread, pasta, rice, potatoes, chips, bagels, crackers, quinoa, porridge, and oatmeal, to name a few. All starched that you consume will turn into sugar once digested and will hinder weight loss. To follow the keto diet, you will find many delicious substitutes in the grocery stores, such as keto bread, keto pasta, keto rice, and many more. For you start this a sample diet plan you can follow:

Breakfast

- 3 eggs, scrambled, cooked in coconut oil

- ½ onion chopped

- 1 bell pepper chopped

- 1 cup black coffee

Post-Breakfast Snack

- 1 oz almonds

- 1 oz cheese

- 1 cup carrots

Lunch

- 3 oz salmon

- 2 cups spinach

- 1 oz goat cheese

- 1 tbsp vinaigrette dressing

Post-Lunch Snack

- ½ apple

- 3 oz beef jerky

Dinner

- 5 oz ribeye steak

- 2 cups grilled vegetables

- ¼ cup sautéed mushrooms

If this tempts you to start the keto diet, consult with your doctor before you embark on this low-carb, high-fat diet. This diet is never a one-size-fits-all prescription. Hence, you must consult with your dietician to ensure you are getting all essential nutrients while maintaining ketosis.

Disadvantages of Keto Diet

Despite the diet's proven results, you will also find many contradicting views about the keto diet. You will find both kinds of nutritionists, some that emphasize the benefits associated with this diet plan and others who recommend avoiding it at all costs. Therefore, if the keto diet is your weight loss solution, you need to be informed about the potential health hazards that come along with it. Following a ketogenic diet includes consuming fats while avoiding carbs. Hence, foods such as butter, cheese, and fatty meats become an integral part of your meals. This causes an increase in your body's cholesterol levels, consequently raising the level of LDL cholesterol, which is unsafe. A high rise of LDL in the bloodstream is particularly more alarming for people with a history of cardiovascular diseases. Therefore, you should get yourself examined regularly or consult a nutritionist or dietician to help you choose healthier food options.

The process ketosis, which is used in the keto diet to lose weight can also prove to be risky. During ketosis, the body forms ketones, and excessive production of ketones can make the blood more acidic, resulting in dehydration. Moreover, the keto diet plan allows only certain vegetables and fruits in a limited quantity. As a result, your body is deprived of many vitamins and minerals that you can gain from these food sources, such as fiber and antioxidants.

Since the keto diet's diet plan is so restrictive, some health experts say it is not an appropriate plan for the long term. Keto diet is best when continued for 30 to 90 days and later followed by a more sustainable diet plan. The problem here is that most people start to regain the weight they lost as soon as they go back to consuming carbs. Besides, such restrictive diets also contribute to eating disorders in the future.

Steps to Consider before starting Keto Diet

No matter what you see on the internet, consuming only keto foods does not guarantee the results you are looking for. To get the most advantage of a keto diet, you need to identify your primary goal, whether it is weight loss, muscle gain, improved performance, or improved health. Once you have determined your fitness goal, the next step is to identify the ketogenic diet variation that works the best for your body type and calculate the keto macros (fats, proteins, and carbs) accordingly. Do not skip formulating a keto menu since it will assist you in choosing more nutritious foods and allow you to stick to your keto diet for longer. To progress, it is essential to calculate the calories consumed in a day so make use of an online calorie calculator or a fitness app to easily monitor your progress.

Following these steps will help your body to carry

on with the keto diet. However, to select the correct variation of a keto diet for yourself, I would suggest meeting with your doctor and understand if you do not have any complications that can conflict with the keto diet. Finally, you should always listen to your body and assess your energy levels when following a diet plan.

Chapter 3: Intermittent Fasting

You must have heard of people fasting for religious reasons, but have you heard or seen people fasting for weight loss? As surprising it may seem, intermittent fasting is a unique form of dieting that involves fasting for a few hours. Compared to many other famous diets, intermittent fasting does not focus on specific foods to eat. Instead, it focuses on when you should eat. Therefore, it is not a diet in the conventional sense but would be more accurately described as an eating pattern, cycling between periods of fasting and eating.

Although intermittent fasting is an eating pattern, the main reason to follow it is still the same as other diets; to lose weight. Following an eating pattern that involves fasting helps in losing weight. Perhaps, it is one of the simplest strategies you will come across for shedding off excess weight.

Following intermittent fasting, the main benefit is that your meals are scheduled to receive the ultimate benefit from what you eat. So, if you target a lean body, it is not necessary to follow those demanding diets that require cutting down your calories. Rather, you can shift to intermittent fasting, which helps to maintain muscle mass by following an eating pattern.

The intermittent fasting health trend has been around for decades. If you notice, this trend has been followed by the Muslims every year as a part of their religious ritual for centuries now. Muslims dedicate a whole month for this purpose, refraining from drinking or eating from sunrise to sunset. Hinduism also promotes fasting, but it is not an obligation, instead, it is a moral and spiritual act to purify the body and mind. The fasting routine followed by Hindus is similar to intermittent fasting since they are allowed to consume drinks and water during their fast. Moreover, the Catholic church also recommends this practice for its underlying spiritual benefits. Intermittent fasting, however, is quite unique to the already fasting trend followed by different religions.

The most interesting fact about intermittent fasting

is how its physical benefits symbolically mirror its spiritual one; in the same way that intermittent fasting aids in weight loss, call repair, and combats diseases, it assists in modifying and evolving the soul's priorities. Hence, intermittent fasting has dual advantages, purifying the body and clarifying the soul. I will elaborate further on the health benefits and how intermittent fasting works. But before that, let's understand the underlying spiritual dimension linked to intermittent fasting.

Intermittent Fasting Instills Discipline & Self Control

If you are new to intermittent fasting, it can be tough. During this process, there will be times when you will fail to control your hunger, and at times you might be successful.

Normally we have plenty of choices in terms of food selection, spoiling us for the longest time. Even when we are not hungry, we consume food items that are not healthy, not because we need it, but we want it. Most of the time, we display no self-control and end up spoiling our diet. With intermittent fasting, traits such as discipline and self-control fall into place independently without much effort. Imagine fasting for 16 hours and ending up consuming high-calorie foods. Following intermittent fasting majority of the people would rather choose a meal which satiates the hunger as well as provides the highest health benefits. Hence, if you start to follow intermittent fasting, you will learn self-control and discipline in no time.

Intermittent Fasting Strengthens your Resolve

In intermittent fasting, we deny our body to eat anytime we like and restrict our food choices. It helps us to repel our temptations and cravings and opt for healthier options. While we physically deny the body of its needs, spiritually, we end up being more clear-headed and mindful of our actions. As a result, we are in a better mental space by being in touch with our spiritual needs, making us more confident in our decisions. These decisions are not only restricted to food choices, but also other decisions we have to take daily related to our work or personal life.

To put together, intermittent fasting helps to connect with our body and understand the true meaning of our identity. Once you start intermittent fasting, eventually, you will observe yourself to be more calm, composed, disciplined, and confident than before.

Looking at the generations before us, don't you wonder why we gain weight faster and find it even more difficult to shed weight? The answer lies in our lifestyle change. With the invention of computers and TV, our physical movement is reduced, and the time spent lazing on the couch has increased. Therefore, you and your children now opt for indoors activities that require less movement. Moreover, we stay awake for longer hours to catch up on our favorite shows and end up snacking and consuming more calories. Thus, following intermittent fasting can help to reverse these trends.

The Science Behind Intermittent Fasting

As mentioned earlier, intermittent fasting does not involve food choices or any food list you might have to follow in other weight loss programs. Intermittent fasting simply alternates the periods of fasting and eating without any macronutrient recommendation. Even without any restrictions, it has become the most popular eating trend. Such that it was prominently featured in an article[xi] of 'The New England Journal of Medicine.'

To understand the science behind weight loss in intermittent fasting, we need to be clear about two main terms; fed and fasted. Your body undergoes both these states when you are following intermittent fasting. When you are digesting and absorbing food, your body is experiencing the fed state. Typically, this state begins when you start eating and lasts for about three to five hours until your body digests and absorbs the food you have consumed. Throughout this state, it's hard for your body to burn fats because the insulin levels are high due to eating.

Soon after, when your body isn't processing any meal, you undergo a post-absorptive state that lasts for around eight to twelve hours after your last meal. After this, your body enters the fasted state, during which it is easier for your body to burn fat because your insulin levels are low. Hence, during the fasted state, your body burns the fat that was not accessible in the fed state.

Now let me connect these two terms with intermittent fasting. On a regular day, you consume three meals or six small meals. These meals do not have a long gap of at least eight hours. Therefore, your body is always in the fed state. In intermittent fasting, when you finish eating, your body experiences the fasted state and starts to use the fat reserves to provide you with the energy to go by your day. Albeit you are allowed to take fluids to keep you hydrated in the fasted state.

Mattson, the adjunct professor of neuroscience, says, "Intermittent fasting contrasts with the normal eating pattern for most of us, who eat throughout their waking hours. If someone is eating three meals a day, plus snacks, and they are not exercising, then every time they eat, they're running on those calories and not burning their fat stores."

If you are confusing intermittent fasting with starvation, you are connecting the wrong dots. Intermittent fasting and starvation differ in one crucial way, that is, control. Starvation is the involuntary absence of food for a long time. On the other hand, intermittent fasting is the act of voluntarily avoiding food for health or spiritual reasons and making it a more deliberate and controlled action.

Intermittent fasting can be as simple as fasting for sixteen hours, including nighttime, and consuming food within the next eight hours. Although, this is not the only fasting plan. There are six popular methods available from which you can choose to alter your eating pattern. However, identifying one method will be tough since each one is effective, but it is on you to figure out which one works best for your body.

1. The 16/8 Method

The 16/8 method is the simplest and manageable method of intermittent fasting. This method was popularized by fitness expert, Martin Berkhan, and is also known as the Leangains protocol. Following this method, you will have a window of around eight hours to restrict your daily eating, and the rest of the sixteen hours will be spent fasting. Within the window of eight hours, you can fit it one, two, or three meals as per your choice.

You can follow the 16/8 method by not eating anything after dinner and skipping breakfast. For instance, finish your last meal at 8 p.m. and not eat anything until noon the next day to fast for 16 hours. However, this method can be hard to get habituated to for people who enjoy their breakfast. If you happen to fall in this category, you can drink coffee or other zero-calorie beverages during your fasting period to reduce hunger pangs. The eating pattern is only effective in weight loss when you consume healthy food and refrain from eating junk food during your eating window.

2. Alternate Day Fasting

The name of this method says it all. This means if you normally eat on a Monday, Tuesdays will either include a few hundred calories or 24-hour fasting and then normally eat again on Wednesday and fast on Thursday. This way, the cycle continues for the week, fasting every alternate day. It is advised not to fast the whole day but consume limited calories to burn them for beginners. You will find several different versions of this method; some allow 100 calories on fasting days, whereas some also allow 500 calories. With this method, you might have to sleep on an empty stomach several times a week, so think it through before starting!

3. The 5:2 Diet

The 5:2 diet is the second most popular method in intermittent fasting. Generally, people who want to improve their blood sugar, cholesterol, and weight loss select this method. Following this diet, you should have a calorie intake of 500 for two non-consecutive days each week. You must consume a limited number of calories that you can burn during the day for the rest of the week. Following this cycle of fasting and not fasting, a calorie deficit is created, which causes weight loss. Let me give you an example to understand it better. You can normally eat every day of the week, except Tuesdays and Fridays. You must consume two meals on these two days, with each having maximum of 300 calories only. The British journalist Michael Mosley has popularized the 5:2 diet, also known as the Fast Diet. However, there are not many studies or research available testing the diet.

4. Warrior Diet

The warrior diet is distinctive from the rest of the methods. Ori Hofmekler, fitness expert, popularized the diet. The warrior diet does not involve complete fasting but eating in small amounts of raw fruits and vegetables during the day followed by one huge meal within a four-hour eating window at night. And the same cycle will continue for the week.

5. Eat Stop Eat

Eat Stop Eat method was popularized by fitness expert Brad Pilon. This plan requires you to eat normally during the week, except fast for 24 hours once or twice a week. The fasting period can be calculated from dinner one day to dinner the next day, completing the 24-hour cycle. For instance, you normally eat throughout the week except for Mondays and Thursdays. So, your fasting period starts from the time you finish dinner on Sunday at 7 p.m. and ends at the same time on Monday, completing your 24-hour fast. In the same way, you can fast from lunch to lunch or breakfast to breakfast, as per your choice. During the fasting period, you can only drink water, coffee, and other zero-calorie beverages and avoid all kinds of solid food.

Using this method, you can reach your weight goal, but fasting for 24 hours seems tough, right? You can always start with fasting for 16 hours and gradually move it up to 24 hours, increasing the pace according to your body's response.

6. Spontaneous Meal Skipping

Spontaneous meal skipping does not follow a structured fasting plan. But there is a catch, to reap the benefits of this method, you need to always eat healthily. This method of intermittent fasting is perfect for people who are either traveling on and off for work or for people who are too busy to cook. Following this method, you have the liberty to skip meals whenever you like, be it your breakfast, lunch, or dinner, and then eat normally, controlling your calorie intake for the rest of the day.

These are the six methods to incorporate

intermittent fasting into your routine. However, before jumping on the bandwagon of intermittent fasting, make sure to consult with your doctor. This will help you choose the best method for yourself.

Advantages & Disadvantages of Intermittent Fasting

Similar to other diets, intermittent fasting also has its fair share of advantages and disadvantages. To better understand, let me take you through both of them before you start off with the new eating pattern.

Most people follow intermittent fasting for weight loss, but this is not the only benefit. Along with weight loss, it also aids in boosting your metabolism. The best part about intermittent fasting is that it is much easier to follow in comparison to rest of the diets available since it does not restrict you from consuming certain food items. The continuation is not long-term with other diets because changing your behavior to certain food items is not an easy task.

Moreover, intermittent fasting has many other hidden benefits, such as battling type-2 diabetes. This is possible because the eating pattern followed in intermittent fasting minimizes insulin resistance and regulates blood sugar levels. Research[xii] has also been conducted in this regard which concludes that intermittent fasting is an effective non- medical-dietary practice that shows promising results in treating type 2 diabetes. Other than driving down the insulin levels while fasting, the body also initiates important cellular repair processes. Besides, with intermittent fasting, the blood pressure improves as well as the resting heart rate.

The more apparent advantages of intermittent fasting are the change in your physical performance. Even though you are fasting, this diet helps maintain mass, giving a lean structure, and might provide you with the extra energy to perform better at the gym. Other than this, following this eating pattern also boosts your thinking and memory.

On the other hand, there are also disadvantages attached to intermittent fasting. This diet requires to fast for longer durations which might not be doable for everyone. Halfway through, you might hear your stomach grumbling for food. While some people can fast for longer durations, others might not be able to and may feel dizzy or even faint. Even if you get through your fasting duration, what are the odds you will not end up overeating? If you are restricted to eat for almost 16 hours, anyone can easily end up eating surplus calories, leading to weight gain. In addition, fasting can affect your sleeping pattern as well as your mood to a great extent. Following this diet, your fasting window is far greater than the eating window. Therefore, you might not want to be socially active and attend friends gathering to avoid any kind of food intake.

Fasting can help maintain insulin levels, but it can negatively affect your health as well. For women, longer durations of fasting and not enough food intake can lead to irregular menstrual cycles and potential fertility issues.

John Hopkins's dietitian Christie Williams suggests that intermittent fasting is not for all. According to him, these people should not try this diet:

- Women who are pregnant and breastfeeding

- Children under the age of 18
- People who are already suffering from eating disorders
- People with diabetes and high sugar levels

However, people who do not belong in any of these categories above can try intermittent fasting and reap benefits.

Several studies support intermittent fasting, but there are still many experts and doctors who do not recommend this diet plan. Fasting can be beneficial in the short term, but it also has its downsides. In the long term, intermittent fasting can lead to eating disorders and depression because of improper eating schedules and no social life. Intermittent fasting does not work for everyone, especially for people who are used to having small meals every few hours. For them, fasting can lead to dehydration and low levels of vitamins and minerals in the body, resulting in extreme weakness, fatigue, and low performance at work.

Dr. Ethan Weiss, a cardiologist who has been an advocate for intermittent fasting, now disagrees with his study after practicing the diet for five years. He monitored himself and realized that there are no apparent benefits with intermittent fasting other than normal eating patterns. According to him, participants following intermittent fasting lost more lean mass than fat mass compared to those who had regular mealtimes. Moreover, he believes it is one of those lousy weight loss techniques that will surely help you shed some weight, but it is not the right kind of weight loss.

What You Need to Know

If you are interested in pursuing intermittent fasting, you should be aware of its pros and cons, the health issues that may arise, and the dangers of diseases resulting from this diet.

The availability of intermittent fasting methods makes it easier to choose a method to suit your needs. But research is still ongoing to understand the pros and cons, and studies are still lacking to know if this eating style provides long-term benefits.

Many people have mentioned that it is easier for them to follow this diet since it does not focus on eating particular foods or limiting any products. In contrast, following other diets, understanding the dietary needs a substantial amount of time and requires food prep time. However, with intermittent fasting, they do not have to worry about cooking, macronutrient limitations, or calorie counting.

On the flip side, fasting for 16 or 24 hours can have some serious side effects. You might feel moody, tired, exhausted, and might not be able to perform your daily tasks at work or home. Fasting can also lead to constipation, anemia, dehydration, hypertension, and high uric acid levels in the blood. In the long run, you might also face liver and kidney diseases.

Studies[xiii] have shown that intermittent fasting is efficient in reducing weight, irrespective of the body mass index. They have also termed it as a choice for a healthier lifestyle. The weight loss results from a calorie deficit in our body, where fat is broken down to provide energy. Hence, promoting an improved body composition.

Whereas sticking to the pattern requires a lot of self-control and discipline. These qualities are required in both fasting and eating. While fasting, it is difficult to follow the prolonged zero caloric consumption, and you are bound to make mistakes or break the pattern. Also, after the long hours of fasting, with your stomach growling and extreme levels of hunger, it highly likely to indulge in overeating. Hence, it is not an eating pattern that can be followed for the long term without roadblocks.

With intermittent fasting, many health issues can arise. With the low intake of food, you might experience restless nights and a disruptive sleep cycle. This is not just a myth, but multiple studies[xiv] have also shown that fasting can decrease your amount of REM sleep, which is important for memory, mood, and learning capacity. Hence, intermittent fasting can be critical to your health. Moreover, during the fasting window, you might feel dizzy, tired, and have a low concentration level because the body is not receiving enough calories to provide the energy levels required to be alert at all times.

Although research says that intermittent fasting may

reduce the risk of diabetes, cancer, and heart disease, but depriving oneself of food for an extended period of time can increase the levels of the stress hormone cortisol in the body. If the cortisol levels are high, they will lead to fat storage, which is not ideal if you are trying to lose some weight. Therefore, intermittent fasting negates the positive health benefits by increasing stress. If you decide to try intermittent fasting, avoid overeating once you break your fast and maintain a good quality diet.

Chapter 4: Alkaline Diet

Like other trending diets, the Alkaline diet also claims to improve health, lose weight, and even fight cancer. The alkaline diet was introduced based on research conducted by biologist, Charles Bernard, who studied the effects of the kidneys in controlling the acidity of bodily fluids. The father of the alkaline diet is Robert O Young, who has published numerous books regarding the topic, such as the "pH Miracle." The introduction of an alkaline diet came along with the popularity of other low-carb diets. However, an alkaline diet is not the same as other diets. What is it that differs in an alkaline diet?

The idea behind an alkaline diet, also known as the acid-alkaline diet or alkaline ash diet, is that the food you consume can affect the pH levels in your body. What does the pH level mean? The Potential of Hydrogen (pH) is measured on a scale of 0 to 14. On one end of the spectrum, from 0-6.9, you have acidic, and from 7-14, you have alkaline or base.

You must be wondering how an alkaline diet is connected to the knowledge of the pH scale? This is important to understand the process of metabolism carried out by our body whenever we consume food. Metabolism is the chemical reaction carried by the body's cell converting food into energy. This process can be compared to fire, how it burns but leaves some ash behind. Similarly, when our body undergoes metabolism, the food we eat is not completely absorbed by the body and leaves an ash residue known as metabolic waste. The metabolic waste can be acidic, neutral, and alkaline, altering the blood's pH level.

How does Alkaline Diet Work?

The pH level of the metabolic waste is identified by the foods you consume. If you eat high acid foods, the metabolic waste or ash will be acidic. On the other hand, if you eat high alkaline foods, the ash will be alkaline. According to the acid-ash theory, acidic ash makes you more vulnerable to illness and diseases, whereas alkaline ash is considered protective. Therefore, you can better manage your pH levels through an alkaline diet.

Producing alkaline ash also provides various benefits to the body. Even scientists agree to maintain a relatively alkaline pH of the blood at 7.365-7.4. Maintaining the pH of your blood can help you shed pounds and improve your energy level.

The alkaline diet is highly popular amongst Hollywood celebrities. Stars from Victoria Beckham to Jennifer Aniston and Kirsten Dunst have embraced the diet over the years and swear by it to maintain the perfect body. Moreover, Victoria Beckham has even tweeted about an alkaline diet cookbook in January 2013.

By now, you must have gathered that an alkaline diet works on the idea of changing the pH level of the body, which depends on the foods consumed. The best part about following an alkaline diet is that it does not have many rules to follow, such as the Keto diet. However, in this diet, you will only have to make smarter eating choices emphasizing alkaline ash-forming foods. Other than your eating regimen, habitual behaviors that increase acidity need to be eliminated as well. These include habits such as tobacco use, smoking cigarettes, drinking alcohol, drug abuse, and ingesting coffee or soda.

Other than this, following an alkaline diet requires slight changes in your sedentary lifestyle, such as overdoing workouts and staying dehydrated for longer. These lifestyle practices can also impact the pH level in your body.

Life-Changing Benefits/Promises of Alkaline Diet

If you happen to consume more than three cups of coffee in a day, your body goes into an acidic state. With too much acid in the body, the oxygen supply is decreased to the cells in the body. Therefore, the cell's ability to repair and collect nutrients declines, causing you to feel dizzy and tired throughout the day. The unnecessary build-up of acid in the body makes you feel fatigued and lethargic throughout the day. However, if the consumption of acidic drinks and foods is minimized and replaced with alkaline foods, it will help your body fight fatigue.

Generally, when we do not consume enough calcium, our body uses calcium from our bones to balance the pH of the body and blood. Hence, as we age, our bones become brittle, leading to osteoporosis. The alkaline diet suggests avoiding acidic foods so that dietary acid load does not affect the protein and calcium in the body. Therefore, following this diet, your bones are strengthened, preparing your body for old age. Besides this, an alkaline diet also helps prevent diseases such as arthritis, cancer, and diabetes.

Moreover, if your body has an unbalanced pH, its ability to fight bacteria and viruses is minimized. Therefore, alkalizing is necessary to eliminate the probability of disease and to strengthen your immune system.

What Should be Consumed Following an Alkaline Diet?

To get started with the alkaline diet, there are some tips you can use to stay committed to the diet in the long run. The basic rule of thumb is to include 80% of alkalizing food items, and the other 20% should be acid-forming. This rule applies to every meal, beverage, and snack of the day. The best strategy to avoid acidic food items is to start by filling your plate with plant foods so that there is not much room left for acid-forming meats and slices of bread. Unlike other diets, with the alkaline diet, you do not need to follow a calculator but simply eyeball your food intake to make the necessary swaps.

In an alkaline diet, the food is divided into three basic categories: acidic, neutral, and alkaline. Acidic foods include red meat, fish, poultry, alcohol, chocolate, wheat, dairy, eggs, and grains. The neutral foods consist of natural fats, butter, milk, cream, starches, and sugar. In comparison, alkaline foods emphasize fruits and vegetables such as apples, bananas, avocados, bell pepper, sweet potato, almonds, tofu, lentils, red wine, white wine, lemon juice, and other food items and beverages with an alkaline pH level.

This diet does not have many restrictions, but the main goal of your alkaline diet should be to simply consume more alkaline foods and less acidic foods. Your daily diet should revolve around eating as many fruits and vegetables as possible, along with drinking 64 ounces of water every day. You can even add a dash of lime juice to the water without worrying about lemons being citrus fruits because they have an alkalizing effect within the body.

When following an alkaline diet, you can also add an alkaline broth (vegetable broth) to your daily diet to provide you with all the vitamins and minerals. If you are used to consuming animal protein, you will have to restrict its intake to just one serving each day. Other than this, to reap the benefits of an alkaline diet, it is also required to drink less soda and coffee or eliminate intake altogether.

Side Effects & Cons of Alkaline Diet

Although the alkaline diet reinforces the old-fashioned healthy eating regimen full of fruits and vegetables, no research or scientific evidence supports the claim of the diet, changing the body's pH level. Let us dive into the chemistry of the human body once again. In a natural state, the blood in a human body is slightly alkaline, hovering between the pH level of 7.35 and 7.45. In contrast, the pH level of the stomach is always acidic, maintained at around 3.5, so to help digest the food consumed. Though the food consumed can affect our urine's pH level, this is how our body is functioned to maintain steady pH levels in the human blood. The pH levels in our body are tightly regulated, keeping them constant to carry out the functions. Therefore, nothing you eat can substantially change the pH levels of the body. Thus, the food items you consume following an alkaline diet can only support a healthy weight loss.

Although the diet promotes healthy foods, it also restricts the intake of nutritious foods such as eggs, milk, and other dairy products, which are a great source of protein and calcium. Moreover, the theory that the body absorbs calcium from the bones to balance out acidity has been denied by research[xv] conducted in 2015. It states that dietary acid load has no significant associations with bone mineral density or osteoporosis diagnosis.

Furthermore, consuming only alkaline food products can have an adverse effect on the body, potentially disrupting the body's natural pH balance. If the bloodstream loses too much acidity, there is a higher chance for the body to experience alkalosis. This may lead to hand tremors, vomiting, nausea, and muscle twitching.

Is Alkaline diet a Healthy Choice for You?

Adopting an alkaline diet can highly improve the nutritional level in your body. The plant-based diet promotes incorporating fruits and vegetables in your diet to help you achieve your target weight, overall wellness and protect against certain diseases without any special supplements.

An alkaline diet is easy but can be challenging for many people. If you love to cook and experiment with your food, this diet is best for you. On the other hand, people who are real foodies and travel frequently will find it tough to follow the diet. An alkaline diet completely restricts food items such as meat, bread, and sweets which are allowed in moderation in other diets. In addition, eating out can also be a challenge since food selection according to the diet can be a tight spot.

Not to mentions, this diet does not apply to everyone. People with kidney diseases and gastrointestinal diseases should avoid an alkaline diet since it can negatively impact the body's functions. Especially people who are in the advanced stages of chronic kidney disease are at a high risk of hyperkalemia – high blood potassium levels – that is due to an alkaline diet high in fruits and vegetables. Therefore, if you belong to this group, make sure to talk with your doctor or dietitian before switching to an alkaline diet.

Finally, an alkaline diet promotes weight loss, but you need to factor in exercise in your daily routine like any other diet. It is recommended to incorporate at least 150 minutes of exercise each week. However, before starting any diet, make sure to understand it and consult your doctor for the best results.

Chapter 5: Which Diet to Choose?

One thing that all experts agree on is that the right weight loss plan is one that you can stick to in the long term. Michelle May, MD, author of *Am I Hungry? What to Do When Diets Don't Work*, says, "It doesn't matter how scientifically sound the program is (and many are not), how fast they work (you will regain as fast as you lost), or even how many people have tried it before. What matters is whether you can do what they say forever -- not whether you should, but whether you can."

Of course, not all diet plans and services are backed by factual work. Judy Rodriguez, PhD, RD, author of *The Diet Selector*, speaks, "Just because it is on the bookshelf, or the name is on a door, it does not mean it is a healthy, well-rounded program."

Nonetheless, it appears that the diets that everybody desires are the ones that promise the fastest, pain-free results — which, sadly, are seldom permanent. When you lose weight quickly, it's usually a combination of water, muscle, and a little fat, rather than just fat. Worse still, losing is always accompanied by gaining.

"Most people go on and off fad diets and fall into the yo-yo syndrome of dropping weight followed by gaining weight," states Rodriquez, a professor of nutrition at the University of North Florida. "The consequence is, you lower your metabolism and end up at a heavier weight than when you started."

There is no lack of advice when it comes to weight loss. Mags, journals, and blogs all claim that if you follow diets that reduce fat or carbohydrates or promote superfoods or special supplements, you'll lose all the weight you want for real.

So, how exactly do you know which solution would work for you when there are so many contradictory options? First things first, let's start by analyzing all the different diets and the quirks that set them apart from the others to make an informed choice.

Now, what really is the difference between a

vegetarian and a vegan? What about a flexitarian and a pescatarian? You might also be unfamiliar with the term macrobiotic. Let's take a look.

The Vegan Diet

Meat, fish, poultry, eggs, and dairy products, as well as other animal-derived items like honey, are not allowed on this diet. Rennet, gelatin, collagen, and other types of animal protein, as well as stocks and fats made from animals, are not allowed on this diet.

However, veganism is more than just a set of dietary principles for being healthy. Vegans are also opposed to any product that entails the use of animals for human purposes, whether directly or indirectly. Leather goods, wool, silk, beeswax, animal-tested cosmetics, latex products containing casein (extracted from milk proteins), and specific soaps, and candles made from animal fats are among these goods.

The Vegetarian Diet

All animal flesh products, such as red meat, fish, and poultry, are avoided by vegetarians. It could also mean avoiding byproducts from animals that have been filtered for food. It is also adopted for ethical or environmental reasons, in addition to the health benefits of potentially lowering your risk of chronic diseases.

Vegetarians are divided into a few sub-types:

- **Lacto-ovo-vegetarian diet:** Fish, meat, and poultry are prohibited, but eggs and dairy products are allowed in this diet.

- **Lacto-vegetarian diet:** Fish, meat, poultry, and eggs are prohibited, but dairy products are permitted.

- **Ovo-vegetarian diet:** Fish, meat, poultry, and dairy products are not allowed, but eggs are permitted.

A few vegetarians follow a few vegan practices in their daily lives, such as forgoing products that are tested on animals or made with animal-like leather.

The Pescatarian Diet

With the exception of fish, this diet excludes all animal flesh and meat (such as red meat and poultry). A pescatarian is a vegetarian who eats fish and other seafood such as shrimp, mussels, salmon, crabs, and lobster, along with their vegetarian diet.

Even so, a pescatarian is not a vegetarian; the two diets are markedly different because all animals are excluded from a vegetarian diet.

Beans and legumes, such as tofu and tempeh, as well as vegetables, fruits, grains, and dairy products, are permitted for pescatarians. The moderate consumption of fish or fish oils, which are high in Omega-3 fatty acids and a major component of one's diet, is among the diet's benefits.

The Flexitarian Diet

Individuals who consume veggies primarily but every once in a while eat meat, such as poultry, red meat, fish, and seafood, fall into this category. When they eat meat, they prefer free-range or natural animal foods. They are also known as semi-vegetarians. There is no hard and fast rule about how much meat you should consume throughout the week; whether it's once per day, once every week, or once in a while, the amount of meat you consume is entirely up to you.

The Macrobiotic Diet

The Macrobiotic diet, popularized by the Japanese, isn't only about consuming specific foods. It's also about finding stability in your life through food options. Macrobiotic dieters are encouraged to eat regularly, munch their food thoroughly, keep a check on their body needs, stay active, and keep a positive mindset.

Vegetables, whole grains, and beans are all allowed in the macrobiotic diet. Organically grown whole grains such as millet, barley, brown rice, corn, and oats should account for forty to sixty percent of the diet. Vegetables should account for twenty to thirty percent of the diet (with the main focus on Asian vegetables like bok choy and daikon and sea vegetables, like nori, agar, and seaweed).

Beans and legumes, such as tofu and tempeh, should account for five to ten percent of the diet.

Fresh fish and seafood, as well as locally grown fruit, pickles, and nuts, can also be consumed. Rice syrup is one of the sweeteners that can be consumed occasionally.

Meanwhile, eggs, dairy, red meat, poultry, refined sugars, fruit juice, tropical fruits, and certain vegetables such as eggplant, spinach, asparagus, zucchini, and tomatoes are all avoided by macrobiotic eaters. Everything spicy, as well as hard liquor, coffee, soda, and anything processed, refined, or synthetically preserved, is strictly prohibited in the diet.

This diet even dictates which type of kitchenware should be used (yikes!). Specific materials, such as wood or glass, should be used in the kitchen, while others, like copper, plastic, and non-stick coatings, should be avoided.

One thing is for sure, each of these dietary habits has one common factor: they emphasize whole foods and foods with minimal processing, as well as little added sugar and fat. Fried items, sweets, and other highly processed foods with added sugar and fat are not nutritious nor healthy on a plate.

Tips to Select the Most Appropriate Weight-Loss Plan

We now know all about our options. Having established that, it's time we go over some tips that may aid you in selecting a weight loss program best suited to you.

1. Make your doctor a part of your weight-loss plan

Consult your doctor before beginning a weight-loss program. Your doctor will go through any medical conditions or drugs you're taking that may be affecting your weight and recommend a program for you. You can also talk about how to work out in a safe manner, particularly if you have medical or physical issues or if everyday activities cause you pain. Inform your doctor about your past weight-loss attempts. Be honest about your interest in fad diets. Your doctor might be able to refer you to a registered dietitian or steer you to weight-loss support groups.

2. Take into account your individual requirements

There is no one-size-fits-all diet or weight-loss strategy that will work for everyone. However, if you think about your interests, lifestyle, and weight-loss goals, you'll most likely be able to find a plan that fits your needs.

Consider the following before beginning a weight-loss program:

Diets you've tried in the past. What did you like about them, and what did you dislike about them? Have you been able to stick to the diet? What went well, and what didn't? How did the diet make you feel emotionally, physically, and psychologically?

Your personal preferences. Do you prefer to follow a weight-loss plan on your own or with the help of a group? Do you prefer online or in-person meetings if you do decide on group support?

Your allowance. Many weight-loss plans necessitate the purchase of supplements or meals, as well as visits to weight-loss centers and support groups. Is the price within your price range?

There are some other factors to remember. Have you been diagnosed with diabetes, heart disease, or allergies? Do you have any dietary restrictions or preferences based on your ethnicity or culture?

3. Look for a weight-loss program that is both healthy and reliable

One pound of fat is 3,500 calories, so many calories are needed to lower fat. The quick loss of weight is more fluid than the loss of fat. Although it's easy to believe in claims of drastic weight loss, the experts agree a gradual strategy is easier to manage and typically outlasts dramatic weight loss in the long run. The standard advice to a secure and reliable weight loss is to lose 0.5 to 2 pounds (0.2 to 0.9 kilograms) each week and is best achieved with a daily diet and exercise of about 500 calories. Faster weight loss can be safe in certain circumstances if performed correctly, such as on a very low-calorie diet under a doctor's supervision or during a short quick-start period of a balanced diet plan.

Weight loss success necessitates a long-term dedication to make healthy food, workout, and behavioral improvements. Behavioral change is critical and will have the biggest effect on your long-term weight-loss goals. Make sure you choose a strategy that you can live with. Look for the following characteristics:

Flexibility is a virtue. A flexible diet does not exclude specific foods or food groups but rather requires a wide range of foods from all of the major food groups. Vegetables and fruits, whole grains, low-fat dairy products, lean protein sources, nuts, and seeds are all part of a balanced diet. If you like, you can indulge in an occasional, rational indulgence with a flexible plan. This should include items that are readily available in your local supermarket and that you enjoy consuming. Nevertheless, since the calories in these foods don't have enough nutrients, the strategy should restrict alcohol, sugary beverages, and high-sugar sweets.

Achieve stability. Enough nutrients and calories should be included in your diet. Nutritional issues can be caused by eating excessive amounts of specific foods, such as grapefruit or meat; dramatically reducing calories; or removing whole food classes, such as carbs. Excessive vitamins or supplements are not needed for a safe and balanced diet.

Affability. A diet should also have foods that you love and can consume for the rest of your life, not foods that you can handle for the duration of the plan. If you don't really like the food on the menu, if it's too restrictive, or if it gets boring, you're highly improbable to stick to it long enough to lose weight. The key to losing weight is to avoid feeling that you are on a diet. If a diet makes an individual become obsessed with food, an increased craving can be created, and the urge to throw in the proverbial "towel" can be exasperating. Search for a plan that helps you understand ways in which you can reach a healthy weight.

Physical Activity. Physical exercise should be part of your schedule. Exercising and eating fewer calories will help you lose weight faster. Exercise also has a number of health benefits, including preventing muscle loss that happens as a result of weight loss. Workouts are also essential for weight loss maintenance. Workouts are also essential for weight loss maintenance.

4. What are your choices?

Some of the more popular diets are mentioned in the table below. Although there is some variation, most proposals can be divided into a few broad categories. When comparing various weight-loss plans, researchers discovered that the majority of the result in weight loss was in the short term when opposed to doing nothing. Dietary variations in weight loss are usually minor.

When evaluating weight-loss plans, ask yourself these questions.

Take the time to learn everything you can about a weight-loss plan before you start. It doesn't mean a diet is right for you just because it's trendy or your friends are doing it. Second, ask yourself the following questions:

What's in it for you? Is there any advice on the strategy that you can adjust to your situation? Is it necessary to purchase special meals or supplements? Is it possible to get help online or in-person? Is it going to show you how to make meaningful, safe lifestyle improvements to help you keep your weight off?

What is the diet's purpose? Is the weight-loss strategy backed up by research and science? What qualifications, training, certifications, and experience do the physicians, dietitians, and other staff members have if you go to a weight-loss clinic? Can the team work with your usual physician?

What are the potential dangers? Is it possible that the weight-loss program would affect your health? Is it safe for you to follow the guidelines, particularly if you have a health condition or take medications?

What are the outcomes? How much weight do you think you'll lose? Does the software promise that you'll lose a lot of weight quickly or that you'll be able to target specific body parts? Is it promoting before and after pictures that seem to be too good to be true?

5. Is it enough for my exercise level?

Many programs inspire you to workout often, while others just get you going. Ideas that involve hours at the gym may sound fantastic, but they won't last long if you're a desk-bound person. Choose a program with a training aspect that you can do on a daily basis and work your way up gradually. Choose a schedule that inspires you to do something physical that you like and that you can do, whether it's dancing, gardening, cycling, or just cleaning the house.

6. Would the diet include foods I like, can prepare and afford?

Are there any foods or drinks that you're being asked to consume in a mixture or in amounts that aren't sustainable in the long run? Preparations that involve exotic foods or ample time in the kitchen may be ideal for someone with a lot of time and resources, but they might not work for you. Try to ensure the recipes look delicious and save time.

7. Is it still possible for me to eat my favorite foods?

Several diets include long lists and little space for splurges with 'forbidden' food. Specific foods can cause cravings and binges for some people. However, other people are actually better off removing the "trigger" foods that touch binges.

You will have to find a plan that enables small portions of these favorites if you cannot afford to live without a glass of wine or an occasional dessert. But the more stringent plans might be exactly what you need if you're the sort who won't stop with one or two glasses or bites or two desserts.

The Tricks to Losing Weight

Long-term improvements in your eating habits and physical activity are needed for successful weight loss. This implies you'll need to find a weight-loss strategy that you will stick to for the rest of your life. If you go off the diet and fall back into old habits, you're unable to sustain the weight loss you've achieved. Diets that cause you to feel repressed or starving can lead to abandonment. Even if you lose weight, the pounds will easily return once you stop dieting because many weight-loss diets don't inspire lifelong healthy lifestyle changes.

1. Is it necessary to make minor, steady changes?

Many diet plans call for alterations, while others advocate for "baby steps" — smaller, more incremental changes. Change is hard, and the more changes you have to make, the trickier it becomes. If you're up for a big challenge, aim for a strategy that gradually improves your food and exercise habits.

2. Do You Want a More Versatile Program, or a Set-Routine?

To keep on track, several people choose a diet plan that specifies particular foods and portion sizes. Some even prefer the freedom of making their own dietary decisions. As long as a myriad of nutritious foods—vegetables, fruits, beans, whole grain, low-fat dairy, and lean protein—can work in the diet plan. Make sure that the diet plan enables you to have sufficient food and calories to lose weight without starvation.

Hopefully, these tips will help you select the best diet plan for yourself. And while there may be many, *many* options to choose from, it is vital to take your time in researching and really studying the diet program you're considering. We all may be the same species, but we're still unique in our own ways, and I don't mean that in a cheesy way. Your genetic makeup and the many inherent and environmental factors set you apart from each individual. So what may work perfectly for me might not turn out so well for you. And I'm not just talking about the diet plan failing to reduce weight or not working at all.

Electing the wrong program can be hazardous. I cannot emphasize the seriousness of this enough. You have to understand the risks and dangers involved before committing to anything, especially if it's not for you. The wrong diet can be just as injurious as the right diet can be effective. It can cause severe organ damage, mental illness, or even hormonal imbalance. And there's a very real chance of this damage being permanent if you're unfortunate. One wrong move, and you're out. So instead of deciding just to wing it and taking tips off the internet that may leave you prone to harm, you have to ensure your safety and act responsibly and diligently. Always—first and foremost—go to your doctor or a nutritionist to tailor-make your diet program *for you*.

The reason being that before starting any sort of diet, cautious thought, planning, and analysis of your body needs to be made. And a doctor is just the right person to not only prepare your diet plan but also point out what can go wrong, how to follow it, what are the dos and don'ts while on the diet as well as monitor your health closely to make sure you're on the right path. Of course, even with the best of nutritionists and trainers to cater to you, alongside the best diet plan for you, you *can't* be guaranteed the results *you* want within the timeframe of *your* choosing. You see as I said before, we're all different, and that difference is also of our metabolism and body type, as well as how you've been treating it beforehand.

Do not be discouraged, though. While the particulars of your before may not be exactly stellar, and the outcome, not something you had foreseen, rest assured, you will get to your destination if you put in the hard work and determination and persevere through all the hurdles. Again, it's a slow process, and anyone who promises you better results otherwise is someone you need to ignore. Years of neglect cannot be salvaged in a couple of days or weeks. You didn't exactly get up one morning, looked in the mirror, and turned into a fat version of yourself, did you? You can't expect to look slim and fat-free in a short amount of time the same way. And even if you did end up achieving it somehow, believe me, you will cause yourself horrible damage. Not only on the inside, but also on the inside.

Therefore, the significance behind choosing a diet that will not only work for you long-term, but will also ensure your health to be in prime condition, is something that can't be ignored. Because it isn't just about the diet or gaining or losing weight. It's about walking down the path to improvement and healthiness with a sound body, heart, and mind. So in the end, whatever diet you end up selecting, whether it's something that's quite common or something that was strictly designed for you, you should make the effort of reflecting on your choices, doing your homework on the said program, and caring about your own being more than the superficial need to care for how you might look. Because ultimately, looks aren't everything.

One thing you should always keep in mind is that whether it's weight loss, gain, or sustainability, it is a simple recipe: calories in, minus calories out equals weight loss, gain, or maintenance. The recipe is unalterable by potions, detox rituals, or supplements. So go on and begin this new chapter of your life, and best of luck to you!

———————————

---

i This Is the Best Time of Day to Work Out, According to Science | TIME

ii BYU study says exercise may reduce motivation for food

iii https://www.healthcorps.org/there-is-no-one-diet-fits-all/

iv https://www.cnbc.com/2019/06/22/new-study-shows-theres-no-one-size-fits-all-diet.html

v https://www.ncbi.nlm.nih.gov/pmc/articles/PMC2716748/

vi Long-term effects of a ketogenic diet in obese patients (nih.gov)

vii The effects of a low-carbohydrate ketogenic diet and a low-fat diet on mood, hunger, and other self-reported symptoms - PubMed (nih.gov)

viii [PDF] Low-carbohydrate diets for athletes: what evidence? | Semantic Scholar

ix Ketogenic diets as an adjuvant cancer therapy: History and potential mechanism (nih.gov)

x Ketogenic diet in cancer therapy (nih.gov)

xi
https://www.nejm.org/doi/full/10.1056/NEJMra1905136?query=featured_home

xii Intermittent fasting: is there a role in the treatment of diabetes? A review of the literature and guide for primary care physicians | Clinical Diabetes and Endocrinology | Full Text (biomedcentral.com)

[xiii] https://www.cureus.com/articles/12903-intermittent-fasting-the-choice-for-a-healthier-lifestyle

[xiv] How does diurnal intermittent fasting impact sleep, daytime sleepiness, and markers of the biological clock? Current insights (nih.gov)

[xv] Dietary acid load, kidney function, osteoporosis, and risk of fractures in elderly men and women | SpringerLink